SPEED READING FOR BEGINNERS

START READING AT A SHOCKING PACE NOW

Disclaimer

What You Will Find In This Book?

Don't you wish you could read the morning paper faster than you are reading these days? It would definitely get you to work more quickly every day. What about the lengthy distracting emails at work that you must refer and correspond to immediately? Or what about taking the usual fill of bulky textbooks to prepare for your school examinations?

Why use up your hard earned money to extensive and expensive training courses when speed reading is easily a skill that you can teach yourself. In *Speed Reading for Beginners* there is a comprehensive guide to the good and the bad of speed reading. It goes with consideration of people and their own separate set of skills and speed of reading.

Time being the most precious and non refundable of all resources determines your success in life depending on how you use it.

The *Speed Reading for Beginners* eBook contains the following:

1. The average statistics of how much an average person reads.

2. The full comprehensive guide on how to speed up your reading.

3. Comprehensive tips on the techniques that improve your speed reading pace.

4. The various speed reading methods.

5. The Lead In to whether speed reading really helps in the real world.

6. Evident Benefits of Speed Reading.

Just flip the page and start your brain training for superfast reading skills!

Contents

The Lead In To Speed Reading

Reading involves the three essential functions of your eyes, mouth and brain. Your eyes and brain communicate the meaning of what is written but it is the pattern of your everyday speech that determines your routine reading pace.

According to the website of 'University of Utah School of Medicine', speed reading can result in even greater comprehension of context than typical reading skills derive.

When you read in your mind's eye you are speaking words to yourself out loud. You do that because in school you were taught that if you are lagging behind on your reading skills, read it all out loud. The problem with this method is that it slows you down. Don't get this wrong. It's perfect for beginners. According to corporate blogger Brett Nelson, you should not be reading the words you should be *inhaling* them. This can only be done if you start by seeing instead of vocalizing every letter in sight.

The Throwback on Earlier Education

Now for most people who have gone on their entire life via this method the hardest things would be not to vocalize. It may sound perplexing but here's the basic breakdown. People read at the speed they talk while successful speed reading involves reading at the pace you think. So basically you have to skip the actual reading step over towards the stage of comprehending the context.

It just does not end with the reading speed. There is the extent of your vocabulary (don't want that to be a bump on the road, coming across a word that will take you 3 minutes to look up minimum) and the scale at which you are already familiar with the subject matter (remember those rich accented men in suits brushing their words at you and then switching back to corporate numbers like it's everyday jargon?).

Seeing Is Believing

Before the 1920's it was notably said that fast readers were the ones who moved their eyes around faster on the page on words they could fully grasp. But let's make it simpler, speed reading involves your view of the page for one. You could try expanding your vision and comprehend the sentence structure of more than one word by a single glance. Or there is another way in which you expand your vision horizontally on the line and vertically on the following line to comprehend the entire meaning of the sentence.

Start From Scratch: What To Do?

You can warm up by reading blogs. There is always one that you bookmarked somewhere to read later on. These are shorter and may help you take your own test. If not then switch to newspaper stories. The best way to really begin your speed reading is by reading magazine articles. The reason is because they comprise of simple vocabulary and so in the beginning you can practice without that unpredictable factor in the text. For an average adult at 300 words comprehended per minute it would take an hour and 15 minutes to read an entire standard magazine. Challenge yourself to beat this mark now!

Remember the real speed reading guide is yet to follow; you are still sizing your abilities and testing yourself first. So while you are warming up stick to your newest reading speed ratio and apply it every week to the weekly issues.

Now set a goal to read a book this month and make sure it is nothing that you have been procrastinating from reading. Odds are you will end up not reading it any time this month either. A wise move would be to pick something out that you cannot wait to brag about at work or a cocktail party. Helpful tip: prioritizing and pruning helps. If you are fluctuating around 300 words per minute then to finish a book in a month you need a minimum of 11 minutes, assuming the book has 100,000 words. Adding to that the usual reading material that you might come across on a daily basis like how to guides or a school book (if you are a student); the book reading time may leave a dent of an hour and 38 minutes in your schedule.

Words Do Not Win.

Let's move on. In order for this warm up exercise to be effective and not in vain, do not forget to take into consideration the texts, emails and online discussions that you receive on a routine basis. If you are timing yourself then you are already climbing the ladder to more words per minute. Remember if you really want to keep up with your new reading pace, seclude your own time for reading. Do not pick up a book while sitting with the family at the same time. Forced focus does not make multitasking possible.

Many are able to reach 600 words per hour by keeping up training with this exercise. This cuts down an additional hour of reading which literally gives you an extra day's reading every week. It is important that you mentally acknowledge that not all comments, paragraphs and threads are worth your time. The whole point is to comprehend what you are reading; if something does not contribute to that or strikes you as filler, skip it.

Why Would I Ever Want To Speed Read?

Remember first grade where you had reading contests to see who reads the fastest. It was childish then, but right now it may prove to benefit you. Whatever discipline you may specialize in, speed reading ultimately increases your chance of efficiency. This increases your productivity, which in turn improves your chances of success. Texts and words will always be around you, no field of work can minimize or get rid of that for you.

Skeptics say that speed reading should be effectively used when going through newspapers, research journals, magazines, online blogs, etc. The point is that texts whose purpose is to convey a key idea are meant to be comprehended thoroughly.

Speed Readers Are Made Not Born. Right?

A successful speed reader is one with a vast vocabulary and comprehension skills. According to an online test it is difficult for the average adult to quickly read stuff involving poetry and even religion because their comprehension level takes time. The vocabulary may have infrequently or had never came across such abstract concepts. The bottom line is that there needs to be a non interrupted flow of comprehension when speed reading because there is no other miraculous way that can ensure that.

Practice Makes Perfect

Nobody's ever perfect so there is always room. The Western Michigan University's academic resource centre recommends that you start by grouping 4 words first. Then the next four. If you keep this up then the time you devote to reading every individual word is transferred to reading four and the math would suggest it would theoretically make you four times faster to finish reading something that usually took a huge chunk of your daily schedule.

This will come in handy when you are going through several research journals or some business proposals.

The Problems with Speed Reading

The University Of Central Florida claims that most problems with speed reading stem from the quality of human memory. This in no way means that the human memory is directly linked with the pace a person can maintain while reading. Even with improvement of memory, speed reading will not automatically improve. The bottom line is that speed reading is all for naught if you cannot remember what concept you just read through. Slow reading does not necessarily achieve a deeper understanding, just because you are spending ten minutes to dissect the information in front of you. That is the very skill upon which speed reading stands. An ineffective memory is probably caused by poor concentration. This book is supposed to help you perform a self diagnosis of yourself. Some symptoms of lack of concentration that may hinder effective speed reading are listed on the following pages.

Day Dreaming

This is true for many. You always catch yourself day dreaming when faced with a lengthy text. Now if you are annoyed by your own day dreaming and have no clue on how to stop it try this neat trick: every time you catch your mind wandering away mark an X on a piece of paper. Surprisingly this really works. According to many college and high school students this one simple trick psychologically helps them reduce their usual day dreaming.

Blue and Don't Know What to Do

You can never concentrate when you are religiously devoting your time to worrying about things that you cannot fix on the spot. This is more common for college students. Next time you are supposed to speed read and everything that seems to bother you invades your thoughts, just write it down and promise yourself that you will look into it later but not now. This is your worry list. Now to stay true to this method and help the technique help you later on too, you must DO SOMETHING ABOUT THE PROBLEM LATER ON!

Forgot What I Read

Coming back to memory function; if you believe that whatever you are doing is distracting, but you clearly eliminated all potential concentration problems, then it is time to review your environment. Visual distractions are a huge factor to mingle in your memory focus too. It is not always just an auditory disturbance that does that. First off (and this book should not even have to say this) get rid of all types of auditory equipment like radios, stereos and TV. Unplug the iPod (no it does not help you concentrate, that is just an urban myth created by marketers). If you going to read something lengthy, transfer yourself where it is very quiet and it seems like it would stay that way for a while. Any potential for noise is a distraction too.

Now for the visual distraction, you can start by removing all pictures, objects and souvenirs that will make you think about where it came from (because that is what souvenirs are meant for). Now it is always recommended to add something in front of your width of vision but in the case of speed reading you don't need to rest your eyes from the page every five minutes do you? No you want to get the job done so its best if you stay away from the desk facing the windows. A harsher version of this would be to find a place of study that is boring and plain enough to boost the status of your text book to 'fascinating'.

My Mind Does Not Want To Read; You Can't Make Me Do It

Artificial interest can always be created in something even when you are not interested (so take off your whiney shoes). It is your job to do whatever it takes in order to achieve your objective. But it is true that not all reading material is always as interesting and this could be a huge letdown when you are willing yourself to speed read.

Pique Interest

To artificially create an interest in reading something, mentally list the things that are reasons for you personally to read and learn what you have at hand. This could be associated with friends, class fellows, teachers and your own mind. If you want to be extreme think about the future. If you are a college student, envision yourself and what you might be doing linked to speed reading after you graduate. If you are doing a job think about your success rate in the coming time. If this is too raw for a motivation factor, form a discussion around the relevance of the subject to your career or life after you graduate or another way to boost motivation is to opt on being positive. Think of everything as a chance to learn something new. You may not need what you are learning now but think of the time when you might. Plus a mindset where things have to be interesting for you to engage with them is never going to get you anywhere.

If you have ever tried out a balanced healthy diet you will know what it is like. All you need to do is incorporate the same attitude you would have with something you had to eat whose taste never appealed to you but in the end paid off. This will pay off too.

Another trick to motivate yourself is by setting a goal. This will automatically eliminate the reason of interest because now you are not reading for interest. Reading the whole thing has just become a means to an end for you.

Eat Right

It may sound a little strange but what you eat or do not eat affects your concentration. When you have too much caffeine and foods rich in sugar for the whole day or just for the morning. You will notice how your ability to read and concentrate reduces. You will readily welcome distraction so your mind will keep on jumping to different scenarios.

Not to sound like a typical nutrition preacher but a good diet will keep your brainy cogs in motion. You have a better chance at making an effort to motivate yourself. You could try a combination of whole wheat, butter, peanut butter, egg, milk and fruit or fruit juice. Notice how differently you may perform.

Developing Vocabulary Set

Before you embark on the journey to speed read it is vital that you expand your vocabulary. You cannot afford to skip this step as an underdeveloped vocabulary naturally shrinks the chances of comprehensive speed reading.

So to improve your vocabulary bank take heart in the following methods that aid in this.

Flashcards

This is the easiest technique. You are supposed to jot down the words that you think you have to look up and compare this to the sentence once you have found the meaning. Everyday exercise your mind by recalling as much of the meaning as possible from your memory. If you still doubt your memory use these new vocabulary words in your everyday writing materials like essays, exams, performance reports, etc.

Invest In a Thesaurus

This is an essential reference book and should not be used in place of a dictionary. Using a thesaurus to keep track of the words you do not fully understand the meaning of helps you build on the implied meaning in context. It also helps to get you aware of several more words that have similar meaning and those that you might not be familiar with. This is a faster technique with dual word benefit.

Add the Jargon to Your Vocabulary

There is a secret to speed reading in your line of work or if you're a student your course of choice. You see the documents and texts related to what you are working on will be filled with different technical words related to the discipline. The sooner this unique vocabulary is grasped the easier it will become to speed read.

The Implications of Words

It is not just about having a good vocabulary set for the language. You need a custom vocabulary for whatever you think you read the most and would like to speed read to boost your efficiency. For instance the word "theme" may mean several different things in several different contexts or education courses.

Reading Flow Is Not Necessarily a System

Systematic reading is the secret to speed reading. One of the best ways to practice speed reading is through reading a textbook. Now before you start reading you need to form a mental system of reading the book. This is not a question about your basic reading skills but how you will approach reading the content and the sequence in which you will comprehend it.

This is a fancy way of saying that there are in fact effective shortcuts to reading any text at hand. Many scholarly experts have developed methods to improve the way you can efficiently scan through text books. However these systems include qualities of a skilled reader along with the "shortcuts". These were mainly developed to help college students, and many of them have successfully benefitted from them.

SQ2R

The SQ3R stands for Survey, Question, Read, Recite and Review.

1. Survey

First off you can easily pull this off by just looking for the hypothesis for the main concept in clues such as the headings, subtitles, bold words, etc. This increases the potential of understanding as you acknowledge the sequence of topics you get an idea of where this is going.

After this is the time when you need to start speed reading (which will of course become easier because you are almost there when it comes to comprehending the text).

2. Question

Once you have entirely read the contents of the reading material, start making questions of the key idea. Now the ideology behind this step is the infamous 'reading for a purpose' which you will be utilizing when you start forming the questions. Your mind makes it its purpose to find the answers to these questions which automatically triggers the brain to mentally recite what you just read. It does not matter if the questions were answered or not.

3. Recite

For effective speed reading this needs to be done mentally but if you feel you still haven't grasped the concept then you may read the text one more time.

4. Review

This is almost repeated recitation only now your mind does not care exactly what you read but what the author meant to say.

Ehhh....I Got Nothing

A blank mind has happened to the best of us. This is entirely normal. What happens is that you read something and reread it and read it again and again but cannot understand a single word or recall anything. This is an ancient problem so it did give birth to simple techniques for solutions.

The most basic method involves making small note cards and dividing the key concepts in these by just jotting them down. Now just read them out loud. Now since we are on the topic of speed reading so the technique will fork from the original technique. Simply, ask yourself questions relating to something personal and thus without even reciting the text once or twice in your head or out loud you will remember the meaning of the text because the questions will keep on popping in your head when the topic is approached mentally.

The Gear Range for Different Reading Materials

Journals

These are just meant for research. All you need to do is look out for the keywords (to spruce up your vocabulary). This goes to show that no matter how thick a stack of the journals look, they should be read very quickly.

Novels and Newspapers

The best part about newspaper and fictional or nonfictional novels is that they don't require that excellent a memory to function and still can convey the message without the need of total recall of the context. This clearly goes to show that news pieces and novels should be read much more quickly than research journals.

Textbooks

Reading textbooks is the toughest and the best way to practice speed reading. Mainly because they have relatively less common keywords and mostly because you read textbooks to grasp a concept from scratch which means reading a textbook and ultimately comprehending it needs your most undivided attention.

Usually you need to read the chapters in a textbook twice or thrice. But when the textbook speed reading skills are excellent you may do great at comprehension by only going through it once.

Reading Between The lines- Literally

The peripheral vision needed that allows you to read a group of words together at one time can be done if you extend your vision to two lines above or below at the same time. So basically it is like reading chunks out of the text. It involves you not directly looking at the words.

Now on the example below just focus on the dashes above the sentences and see how much of this you can read by sharing your vision on the words and dashes at the same time.

-   -   -   -   -   -   -   -   -   -

After reading / the guidelines / described and shown / in the book

-   -   -   -   -   -   -   -

Anyone will / be capable of / mastering all reading tasks

-   -   -   -   -   -   -   -

At the point / of being the / most skilled speed reader

This is called phrase reading. You can develop these skills by reading magazines and newspapers. Their simple context and small font are perfect for beginners.

Alarm Clock Reading

For this ignore what was said before about technical text reading. Take up something easy and interesting; that is very important because you don't want to be half asleep in the middle of the exercise. A simple paperback novel would a good choice.

Start by taking up nonfiction material.

The Second step would be to promise yourself to work at it and not cut corners.

The third step is to set an alarm timer for 15 minutes. This means you have a reading time span of 15 minutes only.

Since there are no key words, read the book as fast as you can. Sprint through the common words you know from everyday conversation. To motivate yourself think about all the hefty test time deadlines you had to meet in school.

Next when the alarm clock finally rings, (this is most important) count the number of pages you have read and close the book. Remember do not count the words, no matter what.

Speed reading cannot work effectively without your memory function recalling what you read at the very end of it all. Remember the best way to practice this is to paraphrase out loud everything that you read. This way you will realize what you remember and what you do not. Even after the successful speed reading record.

Now prepare yourself for another speed reading and recall session. Only this time you have to make a run for the words. This is done so that you don't make a habit of the singular reading pace in both soft reading material and extremely technical one, so the wisest thing would be to push yourself from the beginning.

Now repeat the process of recall and compare the time duration with the number of pages read.

Guiding the Eye

Your vision is your number one sense when it comes to reading. The first step in using this sense in speed reading involves that you follow the words with your fingers. As children we are taught to do this so as not to lose focus from reading. This is effective to keep you from day dreaming too.

Try keeping up with the pace of your finger and then speed up your fingers pace too. You know that it is effective once your reading comes into sync.

What to Do - The Technique

Determine Current Speed

Beginners should start out by timing their normal and everyday reading speed. Record how many words you can read at one time. A better way would be to take an online speed reading test that will do the timing for you. Plus these sites also have comprehension tests so you do not have to assume that your speed reading was in theory completely understood. Now no matter what you are reading and even though your mind is conscious of the goal of speed reading, remember this test is for when you are normally reading so don't pick up the pace at all for this otherwise there won't be a different record for your speed reading.

Zero Distractions

A lot of people think they read better while listening to music or when they are in a crowded place. However you think you perform best, get rid of it for now. Turn off the TV, iPod and your cell phone. If you cannot find any solitary place then use earplugs when reading.

Don't Know What To Read

Remember all speed readers adjust their pace according to the reading material they have at hand. Refer to the *gear range for different reading material,* which will give you an idea of how you need to approach each text.

Learn To Distinguish

The truth is that all reading materials are filled with notes. Half of a book you can just skim over or just give it a quick look. With practice you will be easily able to acknowledge the pattern of key ideas from fillers.

Speed reading is not performed in a single sprint. You need to realize that skim reading involves you reading the fillers with one look and then slowing down, but only just a bit at important ideas so that you do not have to re read the whole thing again.

Don't Look Back

Train your vision not to go back to the text you have already read. This can easily be done by taking a blank card and shifting it along the text that you have already left so that even if your eyes linger back to the words unwillingly, the card will hide the words reinforcing the mind that the effort is useless. The speed of you dragging the card will also be a clear indicator of your change in speed.

Stop Echoing The Words In Your Head

Stop speaking out the words in your mind's eye. Many people either mouth the words they read or whisper them under their breath to keep focus and comprehend better. Reading the words loudly in your head actually slows you down. What you need to do is comprehend them not read them. Understand the meaning of the phrase before you get a chance to individualize each word and its spelling. Basically you are training your mind to skip a step.

The Finger Is The Best Tool

If you cannot stop the habit of moving your lips in between intervals of speed reading, just place a finger on your lips and keep your mouth still while you read.

If you think your vision is getting confused because of skim reading and you end up glancing back to the same line or three lines below, use your finger. Seriously, just guide your finger through the whole thing and this will give your mind a sense of actually reading everything that brushed by your hand and you won't doubt if you left anything out.

The best part about this technique is that your eyes have an instinctual habit of following motion so it may be possible that they start picking up the speed to read in the same pace as you move your finger.

Widen Your Gaze

When you move on to the next sentence your eyes automatically take the same amount of time to go back the length of the sentence onto the next line. Try avoiding this by automatically widening your vision so that two lines are coupled together.

This technique however needs extreme focus and practice to stay consistent so again, get rid of distractions!

It takes a while for our brain to give every word shape. You need to teach yourself to remove this habit; read 3 to 4 words at the same time and then quickly recall the meaning of the sentence or phrase instead of each word at a time. Your subconscious has the capability to comprehend what was said even if you cannot remember the exact words that were used.

Do Not Give Up

Speed Reading can prove to be a game for you. Practice, practice, practice! Push yourself to the limits of your comfort level and don't give up. If you find yourself making the mistakes you should avoid which means that you have to start the whole thing again. Do it! Don't waste any time brooding over it because before you know it you will be picking up great speed soon.

Time Yourself; Know Yourself

Remember you need to time yourself regularly; otherwise you will not be able to compare your performance and pick out any extraneous variables in your reading methods which prove to be individually helpful to each speed reader. Plus, it works as a positive reinforcement when you start seeing the difference and improvement in your performance and feel that yes you made a difference. So don't forget to reward yourself too.

No Time For Idle Choosing; Keep It Simple Stupid

As a beginner your speed reading session could be around 20 minutes. Take only one book with one crystal clear purpose of comprehending it. Taking up 3 or 4 books, choosing 1 and then switching because the first one bored you is a time consuming and distracting task for the mind itself and can be a huge hindrance in one of your everyday practice sessions.

Set your reading priorities. You could be reading for pleasure and want to speed read because your tight schedule does not allow a colossal reading session which is your favorite thing or you could be reading for information but the huge stack of books and papers drive you to the edges of nausea. In either case your priority must be to find the hidden message the author is trying to convey.

Tips and Tricks

Turning the Pages

Speed readers once reach a goal of words per minute go about practicing other techniques that may not hinder or better their speed reading practice. There is no hard and fast rule about this, In fact there is no magical technique but according to many skilled speed reading experts say it is best if you save on those seconds mainly because you need to not break your concentration and secondly in speed reading every second counts. The best you can do is to wet your thumb and be prepared to quickly flip the pages; eventually you will turn it into an unconscious habit.

The Posture

This is really a serious thing to follow. Sit in an upright position. Experts suggest that when you sit in a comfortable spot on the couch or when you sit slouching you are in the perfect position to slow down your reading, relax and doze off.

Are we there yet? - How to Improve On the Existing Speed Level.

For many students it is a fact that they already have a mental goal on what they want to learn. Especially if they are out of time. The best thing to do here is to check the table of contents and look for the heading that matches with what you want to learn. Basically the first step is to eradicate the topics that are in theory useless to your purpose and point out the texts which are important to you.

Now the next up you need to figure out how your visual eye that guides you to read can eliminate structure words like 'a' and articles like 'the'. These are vital in creating and connecting sentences but when you are practicing and preparing your mind to speed read it is easier if you make a mental note to first eliminate these words. You will be surprised how much of the text you may have reduced. Just skip them as your eyes glances by them. You will know automatically without the 'a' whether it's a plural or not.

Speed reading involves you 'inhaling' all information. You might be very good at speed reading after all that practice but remember you are no good at absorbing or comprehending any details unless you are entirely focused. Being distressed or worried about something hinders this. This does not however in any way mean that your skill has perished. You simply must first find a way to force your focus. Refer to *The Problems with Speed Reading* above and know that it is of no use if you keep challenging yourself to focus with stress barring your brain.

When one learns something for the first time it is always difficult; because to you right now it is something that you may never be able to achieve. However, as time goes by you will be able to learn something that you never could do before. At this point you need a new objective. As a speed reader record again how fast you are currently able to read each minute. Now push the figures by a bit, not too much but remember by the minute, and not number of words or pages because you are past that point in your current stage. Start reading text that you are used to. This requires tougher training. Think of this as a level up in the speed reading game.

Speed Reading: The Last Word

Speed reading is just the next level after you have learned how to read. Like they say there is no age for learning and thus learning how to read does not end when you are seven. Practicing speed reading is not that hard, mainly because you already know how to read and what you are learning is not entirely alien to you; it is just reinforcing and practicing.

Speed reading is now needed by many people in many professions and students with hectic disciplines. In today's fast paced world speed reading saves you a considerable amount of time and makes your mind prone to comprehending things faster which ultimately makes you sharper.